Endomorph diet cookbook

For women

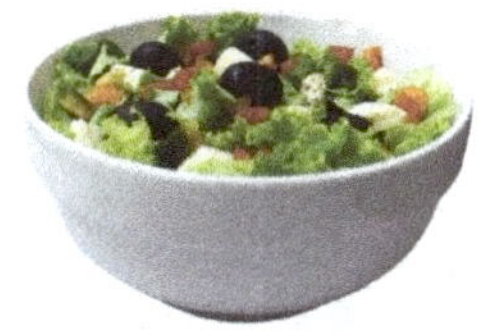

Nourishing and metabolism boosting recipes with a 21-day easy step by step meal plan to fuel your body type

By
David S. Walsh

Table of contents

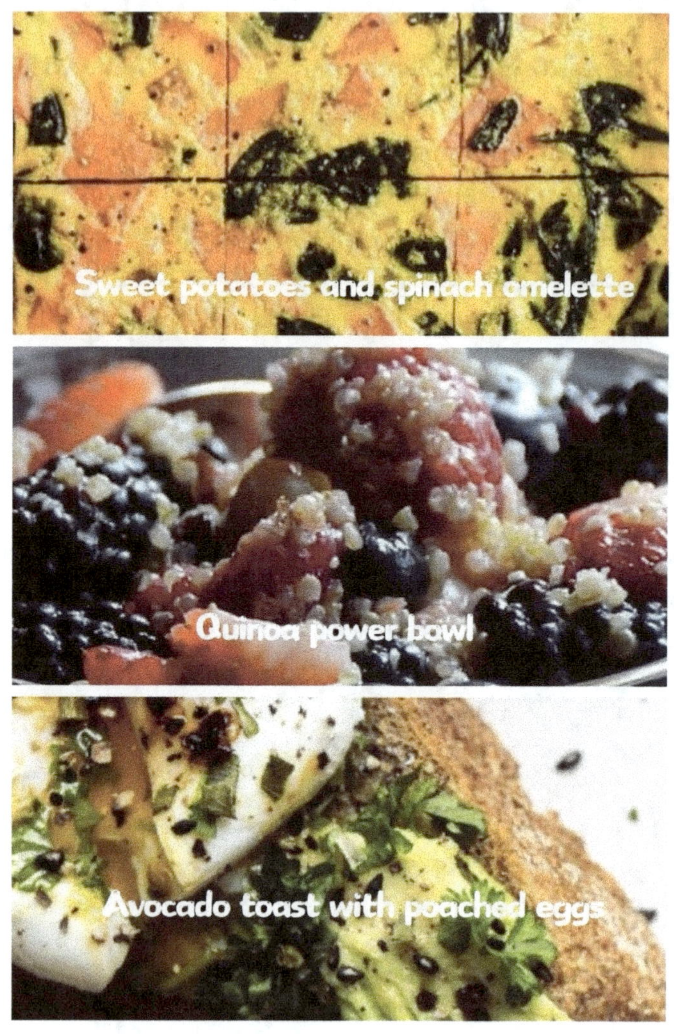

Sweet potatoes and spinach omelette
Quinoa power bowl
Avocado toast with poached eggs

Introduction

In a world obsessed with one-size-fits-all health solutions, there exists a unique and sometimes misunderstood group: the endomorphs. These people, with their distinct body compositions and genetic predispositions, confront problems that go beyond conventional diet and exercise guidance. As a seasoned nutrition consultant, I have seen firsthand the transformational effect of individualized methods for clients embarking on the endomorph path.

Natalie, a determined lady in her mid-thirties who, like many endomorphs, has struggled with weight management despite her commitment to numerous diets and exercise programs. Frustration had become a constant companion until she realized the paradigm change that an endomorph-specific approach could provide.

This book is about more than simply losing weight; it's about discovering one's own potential, accepting the uniqueness of the endomorph body, and navigating a holistic path to health. The benefits go well beyond the numbers on the scale. It's about regaining energy, gaining confidence, and developing a healthy relationship with food.

Before we get into the details, let's understand the endomorph - not as a label, but as the beginning point for a particular trip. We'll look at how genetics shape our bodies and the frequent problems that endomorphs confront. This insight is the foundation of our approach, which recognizes that one size does not fit all, particularly in the field of health and wellbeing.

In the following pages, we'll take a thorough look at the endomorph diet. It is no longer a story of limitation and exhausting exercises; rather, it is one of empowerment and long-term improvement. From the science behind the nutritional principles tailored for endomorphs, each chapter is a step towards a healthier, happier you.

As you read through the next several chapters, imagine a holistic transition rather than just a physical one. This is an invitation to reinvent your story, rethink your relationship with your body, and celebrate the endomorph's unique path. It's a promise of support, advice, and a community of people who share your desire for a better, more satisfying life.

Join me as we explore the endomorph world. Let's flip the page to a healthier, more vibrant self.

Understanding the Endomorph Body Type

In the diverse landscape of body types, the endomorph stands out as a unique group with distinct traits. To really walk the road of health and fitness as an endomorph, one must first understand the subtleties of this body type, including its genetic foundations, typical problems, and the science underlying its composition.

Endomorphs are frequently distinguished by a natural tendency to accumulate body fat. In the somatotype system developed by psychologist William H. Sheldon, individuals are classified into three primary body types: ectomorphs, mesomorphs, and endomorphs. Endomorphs, at one end of the range, have a softer, rounder shape and are prone to weight gain.

Genetics plays an important part in defining body composition, and endomorphs frequently inherit a slower metabolism and a higher risk of storing extra calories as fat. While genetics form the basis, lifestyle choices such as nutrition and exercise have a substantial impact on how these inherited features appear.

Understanding that the endomorph body is genetically inclined to have a larger percentage of body fat does not suggest a set destiny. Rather, it provides significant knowledge, allowing individuals to make educated decisions that are consistent with their specific biology.

Endomorphs face unique hurdles on their wellness journey due to their body type. Weight loss, for example, may necessitate a more deliberate approach, as the body resists losing fat. However, it is critical to debunk the notion that being an endomorph implies a constant fight with weight.

The idea is to adopt personalized lifestyle behaviors that address the endomorphic body's demands. Recognizing these obstacles serves as a basis for developing appropriate food and activity routines that align with the body's inherent tendencies.

To achieve maximum health, endomorphs must learn and embrace nutritional concepts specific to their body type. Balancing macronutrients, such as proteins, lipids, and carbs, is critical. A focus on nutrient-dense meals not only benefits general health, but also assists in efficient weight management.

Endomorph diets require a high degree of customization. What works for various body types may not have the same outcomes. Thus, developing a customized strategy that is tailored to individual tastes, lifestyle, and metabolism is critical.

Certain foods can be powerful allies for endomorphs looking to optimize their metabolism.

Incorporating metabolism-boosting superfoods, such as lean proteins, fiber vegetables, and omega-3 fatty acid-rich meals, can have a significant influence. These options not only help with weight control, but they also improve general health.

Meal preparation is crucial to the endomorph's nutritional journey. Creating tactics that make meal preparation easy and fun promotes healthy eating habits.

Understanding the endomorph body type is not about accepting predefined limits, but rather about gaining knowledge and empowerment. Individuals who understand genetics, common issues, and nutritional recommendations can begin on a transforming path that honors their bodies' individuality.

As we explore the complexities of the endomorph body type, it becomes clear that health and fitness are not one-size-fits-all endeavors. Endomorphs may confidently manage their wellness path by adopting individualized methods to nutrition and exercise, overcoming misconceptions and attaining their health objectives. This insight serves as the foundation for the comprehensive approach we'll take in later chapters, encouraging endomorphs toward sustainable health and vitality.

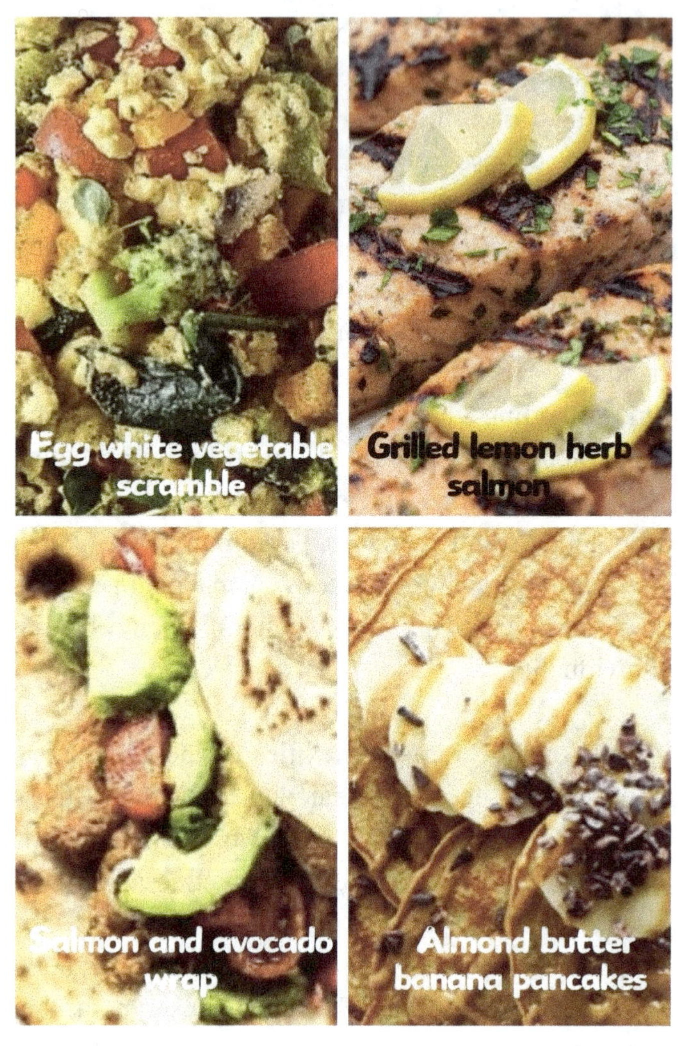

Egg white vegetable scramble
Grilled lemon herb salmon
Salmon and avocado wrap
Almond butter banana pancakes

Chapter 1: Foundations of the endomorph diet

Nutritional Principles for Endomorphs

Understanding and embracing the unique nutritional needs of endomorphs is a crucial step towards achieving health and fitness goals. Endomorphs, who are prone to fat storage, frequently struggle with weight management. However, with a personalized dietary plan, they can not only maintain a healthy weight but also optimize their overall well-being

Macro and micronutrient requirements

1. Balanced macronutrient ratio:
Endomorphs benefit from a well-balanced macronutrient ratio, including proteins, carbs, and lipids. Protein is required for muscle maintenance and repair, while a modest amount of healthy fats, such as those found in avocados and nuts, helps balance hormones and promotes satiety. Whole grains, vegetables, and fruits should be the primary

sources of carbohydrates, as they provide a consistent energy release.

2. Adequate protein intake:

The endomorph's diet is heavily protein-based. It helps to maintain lean muscle mass, which is especially significant because endomorphs are more likely to accumulate fat. Including lean protein sources such as poultry, fish, beans, and lentils in each meal will help you feel full and control your weight.

3. Strategic Carbohydrate Consumption:

Carbohydrates should be chosen carefully. Choose complex carbs that are high in fiber, such as quinoa, sweet potatoes, and oats. Fiber not only promotes digestive health, but it also regulates blood sugar levels, reducing energy dumps and overeating.

4. Healthy Fats for Hormonal Balance:

Incorporate sources of healthy fats into your diet to support hormonal balance. Omega-3 fatty acids found in fatty fish, flaxseeds, and walnuts are very beneficial. These fats promote a healthy metabolism and can help manage inflammation, which is a significant problem among endomorphs.

Importance of Balanced Eating

1. Regular and Balanced Meals

Endomorphs often benefit from a structured eating schedule with regular, balanced meals. This approach helps in stabilizing blood sugar levels, preventing overeating during subsequent meals, and maintaining energy levels throughout the day. Choose three balanced meals and snacks, as needed.

2. Mindful Eating Practices

Endomorphs who practice mindful eating can see significant improvements. Being mindful of hunger and fullness cues, savoring each mouthful, and avoiding distractions during meals all help to foster a better food connection. This strategy improves digestion and can help to minimize thoughtless calorie ingestion.

3. Hydration and Weight Management

Adequate hydration is sometimes forgotten, although it is critical for everyone, particularly endomorphs. Drinking water before meals might help you feel full and avoid overeating. Furthermore, staying hydrated promotes metabolic processes and increases the body's capacity to burn calories.

Diets customized for individual needs

1. Personalized Caloric Intake:
Every endomorph is unique, and there is no one-size-fits-all solution. Adjust your calorie intake to meet your specific demands, taking into account factors like age, physical activity, and metabolic rate. Working with a nutritionist or dietitian can help you find the correct mix for best outcomes.

2. Experimentation and adjustment:
Nutritional requirements might change over time, and what works for one individual may not be suitable for another. Endomorphs should be willing to explore and alter their nutritional strategy. Regular progress checks and potential dietary changes might be critical to long-term success.

3. Consistency over Perfection:
Consistency is key. Instead of aiming for perfection, focus on creating long-term habits. Small, beneficial adjustments made over time can have a huge impact on weight control and general health.

In conclusion, the nutritional concepts for endomorphs concentrate around balance, attentiveness, and customisation. Endomorphs may lay the groundwork for a sustainable and rewarding nutritional strategy that meets their specific demands while also contributing to their general well-being by adhering to these guidelines.

Superfoods for Endomorphs

Understanding your body's specific requirements as an endomorph is critical for developing a dietary plan that promotes health and supports your fitness objectives. One important feature of this diet is the inclusion of superfoods, which are nutrient-dense foods that provide a variety of health advantages. Let's take a look at several superfoods that are specifically designed for endomorphs.

1. Quinoa, The Complete Protein Grain

Quinoa is an excellent superfood for endomorphs since it contains all of the essential proteins. Quinoa contains all nine essential amino acids, giving your body the building blocks it requires for muscle repair and development. Additionally, its high fiber content improves digestion, allowing endomorphs to better regulate their weight.

2. Salmon: An Omega-3-rich Powerhouse

Omega-3 fatty acids are essential for heart health and inflammation reduction, which are particularly important for endomorphs. Salmon, a fatty fish, is an excellent source of these essential fats.

Incorporating salmon into your diet can help boost metabolic function and energy levels.

3. Avocado: Healthy Fats for Long-Term Energy

Avocados can help endomorphs with their energy levels, which are generally low. Avocados are high in monounsaturated fats, which give long-lasting energy without producing blood sugar increases. They also include a range of vitamins and minerals, contributing to general well-being.

4. Berries are antioxidant powerhouses

Berries such as blueberries, strawberries, and raspberries are not only delicious, but also high in antioxidants. These substances assist to battle oxidative stress in the body, which is critical for endomorphs coping with the possible issues of inflammation. Berries are adaptable and may be used into smoothies, yogurt, or eaten as a snack.

5. Leafy Greens: Nutritious Essentials

Leafy greens such as kale, spinach, and Swiss chard are nutritious powerhouses and should be included in an endomorph diet. These greens, which are high in vitamins, minerals, and fiber, help to improve digestive health and supply critical nutrients without adding too many calories. They may be added to salads, soups, or sautéed as a side dish.

6. Sweet potatoes: Complex carbs for sustained energy.

Endomorphs frequently benefit from complex carbs that provide energy gradually, avoiding blood sugar spikes. Sweet potatoes are ideal for this purpose. They are high in fiber and vitamins, in addition to complex carbs. Sweet potatoes, whether baked, mashed, or roasted, are a flexible and healthful complement to meals.

7. Greek Yogurt: Protein-Rich Snacking

Protein is essential for maintaining muscle growth, and Greek yogurt is a great source of high-quality protein. It also contains probiotics that promote gut health, which is very good for endomorphs seeking to improve their digestion.

8. Nuts and seeds: portable and nutrient-dense

Endomorphs can benefit from nutrient-dense foods like almonds, walnuts, chia seeds, and flaxseed. These foods, which are high in healthy fats, protein, and fiber, help to keep you full and may be readily included into meals or eaten as snacks.

9. Turmeric: an anti-inflammatory spice.

Inflammation can be a concern for endomorphs, especially those engaged in regular exercise. Turmeric, mainly its active agent curcumin, is an efficient anti-inflammatory. Including turmeric in your cooking or opting for turmeric supplements can support overall health and recovery

Incorporating these superfoods into your endomorph-specific diet will significantly improve your overall health and fitness journey. Remember that the goal is not just to include these meals, but also to develop a balanced and sustainable approach to nutrition. Experiment with different recipes, maintain consistency, and see how these superfoods affect your energy levels, recovery, and general health as an endomorph.
Fueling your body with the appropriate nutrition not only helps you achieve your fitness objectives, but also lays the groundwork for long-term health and vitality. Accept the power of superfoods and make them your partners on your path to a healthier, more vibrant life.

Chapter 2: Breakfast recipes

Quinoa Power Bowl

Ingredients:
1 cup cooked quinoa
1/2 cup assorted berries (like as blueberries, strawberries, and raspberries)
1/2 cup Greek yogurt
1 tablespoon chia seeds

Preparation Method:
Cook the quinoa according to the package directions and let it cool slightly.

In a bowl, layer the cooked quinoa.

Top the quinoa with mixed berries, distributing them evenly across the bowl.

Spoon Greek yogurt over the berries, creating a separate section in the bowl.

Sprinkle chia seeds on top of the Greek yogurt.

Optionally, you can drizzle a bit of honey over the entire bowl for added sweetness.

Gently mix the ingredients together just before eating, allowing the flavors to combine.

Nutritional Value (per serving):
Calories: Approximately 350-400 kcal
Protein: Around 15-20 grams
Carbohydrates: Approximately 50-60 grams
Dietary Fiber: Around 8-10 grams
Fat: Approximately 8-10 grams
Sugars: Around 15-20 grams (mainly from natural sources like berries and yogurt)

Sweet Potato and Spinach Omelette

Ingredients:
2 eggs
1/2 cup sweet potatoes, grated
1 cup fresh spinach, chopped
1/4 cup feta cheese, crumbled
Salt and pepper to taste
1 tablespoon olive oil

Preparation Method:
In a bowl, whisk the eggs until well beaten.

Heat up the olive oil in a non-stick skillet over medium heat.

Add grated sweet potatoes to the skillet and cook for 2-3 minutes until they begin to soften.

Add chopped spinach to the skillet and sauté for another 1-2 minutes until the spinach wilts.

Pour the beaten eggs over the sweet potatoes and spinach in the skillet.

Allow the eggs to set slightly around the edges, then gently lift the edges with a spatula, allowing the uncooked egg to flow underneath.

Once the omelette is mostly set but still slightly runny on top, sprinkle crumbled feta cheese over one half of the omelette.

Fold the other half of the omelette over the cheese, forming a half moon shape.

Cook for another 1-2 minutes till the cheese melts and the omelette is thoroughly cooked.

Season with salt and pepper to taste.

Nutritional Value (Approximate):
Calories: 350
Protein: 20g
Fat: 24g
Carbohydrates: 15g
Fiber: 3g
Sugar: 4g

Avocado Toast with Poached Eggs

Ingredients:
2 slices of whole-grain bread
1 ripe avocado
2 large eggs
Salt and pepper to taste
Optional toppings: red pepper flakes, chives, or a drizzle of olive oil

Preparation Method:
Toast the whole-grain bread slices to your preferred crispiness.

While the bread is toasting, cut the ripe avocado in half and mash the flesh in a bowl using a fork.

Poach the eggs: Bring a pot of water to a gentle simmer. Crack each egg into a small bowl and slide them carefully into the simmering water. Poach for about 3-4 minutes to get a runny yolk.

Spread the mashed avocado evenly on the toasted bread slices.

Carefully remove the poached eggs with a slotted spoon, allowing excess water to drain, and place one egg on each avocado-covered toast.

Season with salt and pepper to taste. Add optional toppings like red pepper flakes, chives, or a drizzle of olive oil.

Nutritional Value (approximate):
Calories: 400-450 kcal (depending on bread and avocado size)
Protein: 15-20g
Healthy Fats: 25-30g
Carbohydrates: 30-35g
Fiber: 12-15g

Chia Seed Pudding Parfait

Ingredients:
1/4 cup chia seeds
1 cup almond milk (or any milk of your choice)
1 tablespoon maple syrup or honey
1/2 teaspoon vanilla extract

1/2 cup mixed berries (blueberries, strawberries, raspberries)
2 tablespoons almond butter
1/4 cup granola

Preparation Method:
In a mixing bowl, mix together the chia seeds, almond milk, maple syrup (or honey), and vanilla extract. Whisk well to ensure the chia seeds are evenly distributed. Let it sit for 10 minutes.

After 10 minutes, whisk the chia seed mixture again to break up any clumps. Cover the bowl and refrigerate for at least 2 hours or overnight to allow the chia seeds to absorb the liquid and form a pudding-like consistency.

Once the chia pudding is set, take it out of the refrigerator and give it a good stir.

In serving glasses or bowls, layer the chia pudding with almond butter, mixed berries, and granola.

Repeat the layers until you fill the glasses or bowls, finishing with a topping of berries and a drizzle of almond butter.

Serve immediately and enjoy your Chia Seed Pudding Parfait!

Nutritional Value (Approximate):
Calories: 350-400 kcal (depending on specific ingredient brands and quantities)
Protein: 10g
Fat: 18g
Saturated Fat: 2g
Monounsaturated Fat: 10g
Polyunsaturated Fat: 4g
Carbohydrates: 40g
Dietary Fiber: 15g
Sugar: 15g
Vitamins and Minerals:
Calcium: 400mg
Iron: 4mg
Potassium: 450mg

Protein-Packed Smoothie Bowl

Ingredients:
1 cup spinach leaves, fresh
1 ripe banana, frozen
1 scoop protein powder (plant-based or whey, as per preference)
1 cup almond milk (unsweetened)

Toppings: Mixed nuts, seeds (chia seeds, flaxseeds), sliced strawberries, and a drizzle of honey.

Preparation Method:
In a blender, combine the fresh spinach, frozen banana, protein powder, and almond milk.

Blend until smooth and creamy, ensuring a thick consistency suitable for a smoothie bowl.

Pour the smoothie into a bowl.

Toppings:
Sprinkle a handful of mixed nuts and seeds (chia seeds, flaxseeds) over the smoothie.

Add sliced strawberries on top for freshness.

Finish with a light drizzle of honey for sweetness.

Nutritional Value (Approximate):
Calories: 350-400 kcal
Protein: 20-25g
Carbohydrates: 40-45g
Fat: 15-20g
Fiber: 8-10g

Salmon and Avocado Wrap

Ingredients:
4 ounces smoked salmon
1 whole-grain wrap
1/2 avocado, sliced
Handful of mixed greens (e.g., arugula or spinach)
1 tablespoon Greek yogurt (optional)
Lemon juice for drizzling
Salt and pepper to taste

Preparation Method:
Lay the whole-grain wrap flat on a clean surface.

Arrange the smoked salmon evenly across the center of the wrap.

Add the sliced avocado on top of the salmon.

Place a handful of mixed greens on the avocado.

If desired, drizzle Greek yogurt over the greens.

Squeeze fresh lemon juice over the ingredients.

Season with salt and pepper to taste.

Fold the sides of the wrap over the ingredients, creating a tight seal.

Cut the wrap in half, if preferred, and serve immediately.

Nutritional Value (Approximate):
Calories: 350-400 kcal
Protein: 20g
Fat: 18g
Saturated Fat: 3g
Monounsaturated Fat: 9g
Polyunsaturated Fat: 4g
Carbohydrates: 30g
Dietary Fiber: 10g
Sugars: 2g
Omega-3 Fatty Acids: 1.5g
Vitamin C: 15% of daily recommended intake
Iron: 10% of daily recommended intake

Egg White Vegetable Scramble

Ingredients:
4 egg whites
1/2 cup bell peppers, diced (mix of colors)
1/2 cup tomatoes, diced
1/2 cup mushrooms, sliced
1/4 cup red onion, finely chopped
Salt and pepper to taste
1 teaspoon olive oil (optional)

Preparation Method:

Heat a non-stick skillet over medium heat. If using olive oil, add it to the skillet.

Add diced bell peppers, tomatoes, mushrooms, and red onion to the skillet. Sauté until the vegetables are soft, about 3-4 minutes.

Whisk the egg whites until frothy in a bowl.

Pour the whisked egg whites over the sautéed vegetables in the skillet.

Stir gently with a spatula, allowing the eggs to scramble and cook evenly with the vegetables.

Continue cooking until the eggs are fully cooked but still moist.

Season with salt and pepper to taste.

Nutritional Value (Approximate):

Calories: 120
Protein: 24g
Carbohydrates: 6g
Fat: 0g
Fiber: 2g

Greek Yogurt Parfait

Ingredients:
1 cup Greek yogurt
1/2 cup mixed berries (strawberries, blueberries, raspberries)
1 tablespoon honey
1/4 cup granola

Preparation Method:
In a glass or bowl, layer half of the Greek yogurt at the bottom.

Place a layer of mixed berries on top of the yogurt.

Drizzle half of the honey over the berries.

Sprinkle half of the granola on top of the berries.

Repeat the layers with the remaining Greek yogurt, berries, honey, and granola.

Finish with a final drizzle of honey and a sprinkle of granola on top.

Nutritional Value (Approximate):

Calories: 350
Protein: 20g
Carbohydrates: 45g
Dietary Fiber: 6g
Sugars: 25g
Fat: 12g
Saturated Fat: 2g
Cholesterol: 10mg
Sodium: 60mg

Cheese and Pineapple Bowl

Ingredients:
1 cup cottage cheese
1 cup fresh pineapple chunks
1/4 cup chopped walnuts (optional for added crunch)

Preparation Method:
In a bowl, scoop out 1 cup of cottage cheese.

Add 1 cup of fresh pineapple chunks to the cottage cheese.

If desired, sprinkle 1/4 cup of chopped walnuts over the mixture.

Gently mix the ingredients together to achieve an even distribution.

Nutritional Value: (Approximate values per serving)

Calories: 300 kcal

Protein: 25g

Carbohydrates: 30g

Dietary Fiber: 3g

Sugars: 20g

Fat: 10g

Saturated Fat: 3g

Cholesterol: 20mg

Sodium: 400mg

Potassium: 400mg

Almond Butter Banana Pancakes

Ingredients:

1 cup whole wheat flour

1 tablespoon baking powder

1/4 teaspoon salt

1 cup almond milk

1 large egg

2 ripe bananas, mashed

2 tablespoons almond butter

1 teaspoon vanilla extract

Coconut oil (or cooking spray) for oiling the pan

Preparation Method:

In a big bowl, mix together the whole wheat flour, baking powder, and salt.

In a separate bowl, combine the almond milk, egg, mashed bananas, almond butter, and vanilla extract. Mix well until smooth.

Pour the wet ingredients into the dry ingredients and mix until thoroughly combined. Be cautious not to overmix; some lumps are okay.

Heat a griddle or non-stick pan over medium heat and lightly coat with coconut oil or cooking spray.

Pour 1/4 cup of batter onto the griddle for each pancake. Cook until bubbles appear on the surface, then turn and cook the opposite side until golden brown.

Repeat until all the batter is used, adjusting the heat as needed.

Nutritional Value (per serving, makes about 8 pancakes):
Calories: ~150
Protein: ~5g
Carbohydrates: ~25g
Dietary Fiber: ~4g

Sugars: ~6g
Fat: ~4g
Saturated Fat: ~0.5g
Cholesterol: ~20mg
Sodium: ~320mg

Vegetable Frittata

Ingredients:
6 large eggs
1 cup assorted vegetables (zucchini, bell peppers, cherry tomatoes, etc.), diced
1/2 cup red onion, finely chopped
1/2 cup feta cheese, crumbled
2 tablespoons olive oil
Salt and pepper to taste
Fresh herbs (like parsley or chives) for garnish

Preparation Method:
Preheat the oven to 375°F (190°C).

In a bowl, whisk the eggs until well beaten. Season with salt and pepper.

In an oven-safe skillet, heat olive oil over medium heat.

Add red onion and sauté until softened, about 2-3 minutes.

Add diced vegetables to the skillet and cook until they begin to soften, about 5 minutes.

Pour the beaten eggs on the vegetables in the skillet.

Allow the eggs to set at the edges, then sprinkle crumbled feta cheese evenly over the top.

Transfer the skillet to the preheated oven and bake for 12-15 minutes, or until the frittata is set in the center.

Remove from the oven and allow to cool for a few minutes before slicing.

Garnish with fresh herbs before serving.

Nutritional Value (Approximate per serving):
Calories: 220 kcal
Protein: 15g
Fat: 15g
Carbohydrates: 7g
Fiber: 2g
Sugar: 3g
Calcium: 150mg
Iron: 2mg

Oatmeal with Nut Butter and Berries

Ingredients:
1/2 cup steel-cut oats
1 cup water or milk of your choice
1 tablespoon nut butter (almond, peanut, or your preference)
Mixed berries (strawberries, blueberries, raspberries) for topping
1 tablespoon honey (optional for sweetness)
A pinch of cinnamon (optional)

Preparation Method:
Bring the water or milk to a gentle boil in a saucepan.

Add the steel-cut oats and reduce the heat to a simmer. Cook for 15-20 minutes, stirring occasionally, until the oats are creamy and tender.

When the oatmeal reaches your preferred consistency, remove it from the heat.

Stir in the nut butter of your choice until well combined.

Pour the oatmeal into a bowl and top with the mixed berries.

If desired, drizzle honey on the berries for more sweetness.

Add a sprinkle of cinnamon on top for added flavor.

Serve warm and enjoy your nutritious oatmeal with nut butter and berries!

Nutritional Value (Approximate):
Calories: 350-400 kcal
Protein: 12g
Fat: 12g
Carbohydrates: 55g
Fiber: 8g
Sugars: 10g

Whole Grain Breakfast Burrito

Ingredients:
1 whole-grain tortilla
2 eggs, scrambled
1/2 cup black beans, drained and rinsed
1/4 cup salsa
1/4 avocado, sliced

Salt and pepper to taste
Optional: Fresh cilantro for garnish

Preparation Method:
In a non-stick skillet over medium heat, scramble the eggs until fully cooked. Season with salt and pepper to taste.

Warm the whole-grain tortilla in the skillet or microwave for about 15 seconds to make it pliable.

Assemble the burrito by placing the scrambled eggs in the center of the tortilla.

Add black beans, salsa, and sliced avocado on top of the eggs.

Garnish with fresh cilantro for additional flavor (optional).

Fold the sides of the tortilla inwards and roll it up tightly to form the burrito.

Nutritional Value:
Calories: Approximately 400-450 kcal
Protein: Around 20-25g
Fat: 15-20g (mainly from healthy sources like eggs and avocado)
Carbohydrates: 40-45g

Fiber: 10-12g

Vitamins and Minerals: Provides a good source of vitamins A, C, and B-complex, as well as minerals such as potassium and magnesium.

Berry and Spinach Smoothie

Ingredients:
1 cup fresh spinach leaves
1/2 cup mixed berries (strawberries, blueberries, raspberries)
1/2 cup Greek yogurt
1/2 cup almond milk
Ice cubes (optional)
Honey or agave syrup for sweetness (optional)

Preparation Method:
In a blender, combine fresh spinach leaves, mixed berries, Greek yogurt, and almond milk.

If desired, add ice cubes for a colder and thicker consistency.

Blend all the ingredients until smooth and well combined.

Taste the smoothie and add honey or agave syrup if additional sweetness is desired.

Pour the smoothie in a glass cup and serve immediately.

Nutritional Value (Approximate):
Calories: 180
Protein: 12g
Carbohydrates: 25g
Fiber: 6g
Sugars: 15g
Fat: 5g
Saturated Fat: 1g
Cholesterol: 5mg
Sodium: 90mg

Chapter 3: Fish and Seafood Recipes

Grilled Lemon Herb Salmon

Ingredients:
4 salmon fillets
1/4 cup olive oil
2 tablespoons fresh lemon juice
2 teaspoons lemon zest
2 cloves garlic, minced
1 tablespoon fresh parsley, chopped
1 tablespoon fresh dill, chopped
Salt and pepper to taste

Preparation Method:
In a bowl, whisk together olive oil, lemon juice, lemon zest, minced garlic, chopped parsley, chopped dill, salt, and pepper to create the marinade.

Place salmon fillets in a shallow dish and pour the marinade over them, ensuring even coating. Let it marinate for at least 30 minutes in the refrigerator.

Preheat the grill to medium-high heat.

Take out the salmon from the marinade and place on the grill. Cook for about 4-5 minutes per side, or until the salmon easily flakes with a fork.

Serve the grilled salmon hot, garnished with additional fresh herbs and lemon slices if desired.

Nutritional Value (per serving):
Calories: ~300
Protein: ~30g
Fat: ~20g
Carbohydrates: ~1g
Fiber: ~0.5g

Shrimp and Quinoa Stir-Fry

Ingredients:
1 cup quinoa, uncooked
1 pound large shrimp, peeled and deveined
2 cups broccoli florets
1 red bell pepper, thinly sliced
1 carrot, julienned
3 cloves garlic, minced
1 tablespoon fresh ginger, grated
2 tablespoons low-sodium soy sauce
1 tablespoon sesame oil
1 tablespoon rice vinegar
1 teaspoon honey or maple syrup

2 tablespoons vegetable oil
Sesame seeds and green onions for garnish

Preparation Method:
Cook quinoa according to package instructions. Set aside.

In a big skillet or wok, heat up the vegetable oil over medium-high heat.

Add shrimp and stir-fry until they start to turn pink, about 2-3 minutes. Remove shrimp from the skillet and put aside.

In the same skillet, add a little more oil if necessary. Stir in garlic and ginger until fragrant.

Add broccoli, bell pepper, and carrot. Stir-fry for 3-4 minutes until vegetables are crisp-tender.

Return cooked shrimp to the skillet with the vegetables.

In a small bowl, whisk together soy sauce, sesame oil, rice vinegar, and honey. Pour the sauce over the shrimp and vegetables.

Add the cooked quinoa to the skillet, tossing everything together until well combined and heated through.

Before serving, garnish with sesame seeds and thinly sliced green onions.

Nutritional Value (per serving, assuming four servings):
Calories: ~400
Protein: ~30g
Carbohydrates: ~45g
Fiber: ~7g
Fat: ~12g
Saturated Fat: ~1.5g
Cholesterol: ~180mg
Sodium: ~600mg

Baked Cod with Mediterranean Salsa

Ingredients:
4 cod fillets
2 tablespoons olive oil
2 cloves garlic, minced
1 teaspoon dried oregano
1 teaspoon dried basil

1/2 teaspoon salt
1/4 teaspoon black pepper

Salsa:
1 cup cherry tomatoes, diced
1/2 cup Kalamata olives, pitted and sliced
1/4 cup red onion, finely chopped
2 tablespoons fresh parsley, chopped
1 tablespoon olive oil
1 tablespoon balsamic vinegar
Salt and pepper to taste

Preparation Method:
Preheat the oven to 400°F (200°C).

Lay the cod fillets on a baking sheet covered with parchment paper.

In a small bowl, mix together olive oil, minced garlic, dried oregano, dried basil, salt, and black pepper.

Brush the cod fillets with the olive oil mixture, ensuring they are evenly coated.

Bake in the preheated oven for about 15-20 minutes or until the cod is thoroughly cooked and easily flakes with a fork.

Mediterranean Salsa:

In a separate bowl, combine diced cherry tomatoes, sliced Kalamata olives, finely chopped red onion, and fresh parsley.

Mix together the olive oil and balsamic vinegar in a small bowl. Pour over the tomato mixture and toss until well combined.

Season the salsa to taste with salt and pepper.

Serve the Baked Cod:

Once the cod fillets are baked, spoon the Mediterranean salsa over the top.

Garnish with additional fresh parsley if desired.

Serve the Baked Cod with Mediterranean Salsa hot, and enjoy the burst of Mediterranean flavors.

Nutritional Value (per serving, approximately):
Calories: 250 kcal
Protein: 25g
Fat: 12g
Carbohydrates: 8g
Fiber: 2g
Sugars: 3g

Sodium: 500mg

Zesty Lime Cilantro Tilapia

Ingredients:
4 tilapia fillets
2 limes, juiced
3 tablespoons fresh cilantro, chopped
2 tablespoons olive oil
2 cloves garlic, minced
Salt and pepper to taste

Preparation Method:
Preheat your oven to 400°F (200°C).

In a small bowl, whisk together lime juice, chopped cilantro, olive oil, minced garlic, salt, and pepper.

Place tilapia fillets in a baking dish, ensuring they are evenly spaced.

Pour the lime-cilantro mixture over the tilapia fillets, making sure each fillet is well-coated.

Let the fish marinate for about 15-20 minutes to absorb the flavors.

Bake in the preheated oven for 12-15 minutes or until the tilapia flakes easily with a fork.

Garnish with additional fresh cilantro and lime wedges before serving.

Nutritional Value (Per Serving - Assumes 4 Servings):
Calories: 180
Protein: 25g
Total Fat: 9g
Saturated Fat: 1.5g
Monounsaturated Fat: 5.5g
Polyunsaturated Fat: 1.5g
Carbohydrates: 2g
Dietary Fiber: 0.5g
Sugars: 0g
Cholesterol: 60mg
Sodium: 80mg

Spicy Garlic Ginger Scallop Stir-Fry

Ingredients:
1 pound fresh scallops, patted dry
2 tablespoons soy sauce (low-sodium)
1 tablespoon rice vinegar
1 tablespoon sesame oil
1 tablespoon olive oil

3 cloves garlic, minced

1 tablespoon fresh ginger, grated

1 red bell pepper, thinly sliced

1 cup sugar snap peas, ends trimmed

2 green onions, sliced

1 teaspoon red pepper flakes (adjust to taste)

Sesame seeds for garnish (optional)

Cooked brown rice or cauliflower rice for serving

Preparation Method:

In a bowl, combine soy sauce, rice vinegar, and sesame oil. Add scallops, ensuring they are well-coated, and let them marinate for 15-20 minutes.

Heat up the olive oil in a wok or big skillet over medium-high heat. Add minced garlic and grated ginger, sautéing for 1-2 minutes until fragrant.

Add marinated scallops to the wok, stirring frequently, and cook for 2-3 minutes until they start to brown.

Toss in sliced red bell pepper and sugar snap peas, continuing to stir-fry for an additional 3-4 minutes until vegetables are crisp-tender.

Sprinkle red pepper flakes over the stir-fry, adjusting the amount based on your spice preference. Stir in sliced green onions.

Cook for an additional 1-2 minutes until the scallops are cooked through, and the vegetables are tender yet vibrant.

Serve the spicy garlic ginger scallop stir-fry over cooked brown rice or cauliflower rice. Garnish with sesame seeds if desired.

Nutritional Value (per serving, without rice):
Calories: 250
Protein: 25g
Carbohydrates: 12g
Fat: 12g
Fiber: 3g
Sugars: 4g
Sodium: 600mg

Herb-Crusted Mahi-Mahi

Ingredients:
4 Mahi-Mahi fillets
2 tablespoons fresh parsley, chopped
2 tablespoons fresh dill, chopped
1 tablespoon fresh thyme leaves

1 tablespoon fresh rosemary, minced
2 cloves garlic, minced
2 tablespoons olive oil
Salt and pepper to taste
1 lemon, sliced (for garnish)

Preparation Method:
Preheat your oven to 400°F (200°C).

In a small bowl, combine the chopped parsley, dill, thyme, rosemary, minced garlic, olive oil, salt, and pepper. Mix well to create the herb crust.

Pat the Mahi-Mahi fillets dry with a paper towel to remove excess moisture. This helps the herb crust adhere better.

Place the Mahi-Mahi fillets on a baking sheet lined with parchment paper or lightly greased.

Evenly spread the herb crust mixture over the top of each fillet, pressing it down gently to ensure it sticks.

Bake in the preheated oven for 12-15 minutes or until the Mahi-Mahi is cooked through and easily flakes with a fork.

Optional: Broil for an additional 1-2 minutes to give the herb crust a golden finish.

Remove from the oven, garnish with lemon slices, and serve immediately.

Nutritional Value (Per Serving - 1 fillet):
Calories: 220 kcal
Protein: 32g
Fat: 9g
Carbohydrates: 2g
Fiber: 1g
Sugars: 0g
Sodium: 350mg

Cajun Blackened Catfish

Ingredients:
4 catfish fillets
2 tablespoons paprika
1 tablespoon onion powder
1 tablespoon garlic powder
1 teaspoon thyme
1 teaspoon oregano
1 teaspoon cayenne pepper
1 teaspoon black pepper
1 teaspoon white pepper
1 teaspoon salt

2 tablespoons olive oil (for cooking)

Preparation Method:
In a small bowl, combine paprika, onion powder, garlic powder, thyme, oregano, cayenne pepper, black pepper, white pepper, and salt to create the Cajun spice blend.

Pat dry the catfish fillets with paper towels.

Rub the Cajun spice blend generously on both sides of each catfish fillet, ensuring an even coating.

Heat up the olive oil in a skillet over medium-high heat until hot.

Carefully place catfish fillets in the skillet and cook for 3-4 minutes on each side or until the fish is blackened and cooked through.

Remove from heat and let it rest for a few minutes before serving.

Nutritional Value (per serving):
Calories: ~220 kcal
Protein: ~25g
Fat: ~11g
Carbohydrates: ~3g

Fiber: ~1g
Sodium: ~800mg

Mango Avocado Tuna Salad

Ingredients:
1 can (5 oz) tuna, drained
1 ripe mango, diced
1 avocado, diced
1/4 cup red onion, finely chopped
1/4 cup cilantro, chopped
1 tablespoon lime juice
2 tablespoons extra-virgin olive oil
Salt and pepper to taste

Preparation Method:
In a large bowl, combine the drained tuna, diced mango, diced avocado, chopped red onion, and cilantro.

In a small bowl, whisk together lime juice and extra-virgin olive oil to create the dressing.

Pour the dressing over the tuna mixture and gently toss to coat evenly.

Season with salt and pepper to taste.

Refrigerate the salad for at least 30 minutes to allow the flavors to blend.

Serve chilled, either on its own or over a bed of fresh greens.

Nutritional Value (Per Serving):
Calories: 320 kcal
Protein: 20g
Carbohydrates: 25g
Dietary Fiber: 7g
Sugars: 15g
Fat: 18g
Saturated Fat: 2.5g
Cholesterol: 20mg
Sodium: 300mg

Coconut-Lime Grilled Shrimp Skewers

Ingredients:
1 pound large shrimp, peeled and deveined
1/2 cup coconut milk
2 tablespoons fresh lime juice
2 cloves garlic, minced
1 tablespoon of soy sauce (or tamari for a gluten-free alternative)

1 tablespoon honey or maple syrup
1 teaspoon grated ginger
1 teaspoon coconut oil, melted
Salt and pepper to taste
Wooden skewers (soak for at least 30 minutes in water)

Preparation Method:

In a bowl, whisk together coconut milk, lime juice, minced garlic, soy sauce, honey or maple syrup, grated ginger, melted coconut oil, salt, and pepper. This creates the marinade.

Place the peeled and deveined shrimp into a shallow dish or a resealable plastic bag. Pour the marinade over the shrimp, making sure they are thoroughly covered. Marinate in the refrigerator for at least 30 minutes to enable the flavors to integrate.

Preheat the grill to medium-high heat.

Thread the marinated shrimp onto the soaked wooden skewers.

Grill the shrimp skewers for 2-3 minutes per side or until the shrimp are opaque and slightly charred.

Remove from the grill and serve immediately, garnished with additional lime wedges and fresh cilantro if desired.

Nutritional Value (per serving, approximately 4 skewers):
Calories: 220 kcal
Protein: 24g
Carbohydrates: 6g
Fat: 11g
Saturated Fat: 8g
Fiber: 1g
Sugar: 4g
Sodium: 420mg

Lemon Dill Zucchini Noodles with Crab

Ingredients:
4 medium-sized zucchinis, spiralized into noodles
1 cup of cooked and selected lump crab meat
2 tablespoons olive oil
2 cloves garlic, minced
Zest of 1 lemon
Juice of 1 lemon
2 tablespoons fresh dill, chopped
Salt and pepper to taste

Grated Parmesan cheese for garnish (optional)

Preparation Method:
Heat up the olive oil in a large skillet over medium heat.

Add minced garlic and sauté until fragrant.

Add zucchini noodles to the skillet and toss gently for 2-3 minutes until they are just tender but still crisp.

Add lump crab meat, lemon zest, lemon juice, and fresh dill to the skillet. Continue tossing until the ingredients are well combined and heated through.

Season with salt and pepper to taste.

Remove from heat and serve the zucchini noodles and crab mixture on plates.

Optionally, garnish with grated Parmesan cheese for an extra layer of flavor.

Nutritional Value (Per Serving):
Calories: 230 kcal
Protein: 18g
Carbohydrates: 12g
Dietary Fiber: 3g

Sugars: 6g
Fat: 12g
Saturated Fat: 1.5g
Cholesterol: 45mg
Sodium: 380mg

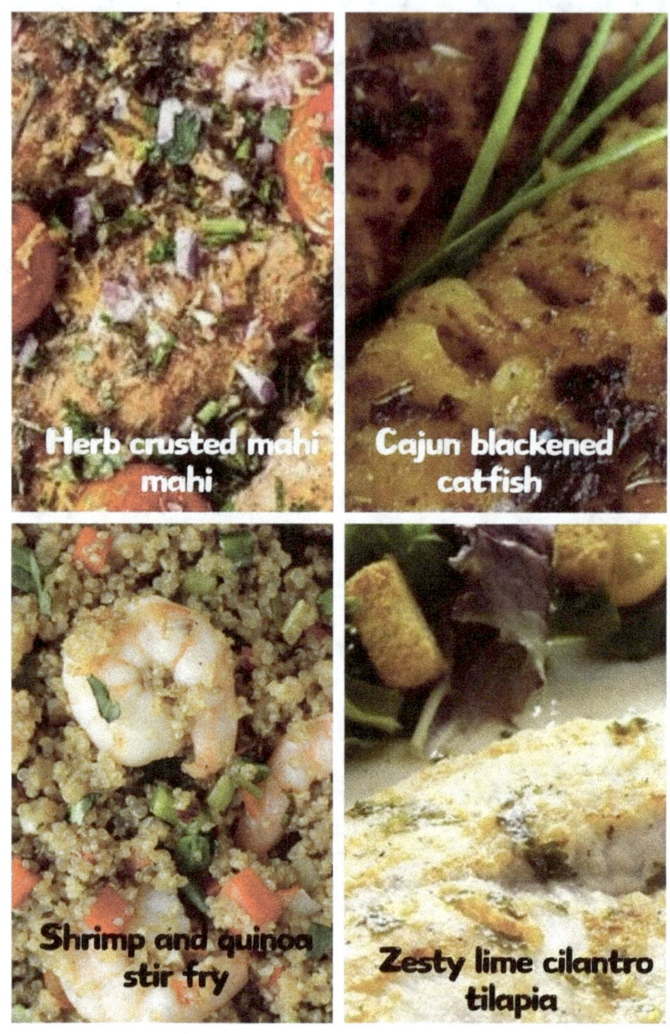
Herb crusted mahi mahi
Cajun blackened catfish
Shrimp and quinoa stir fry
Zesty lime cilantro tilapia

Chapter 4: Beef and Poultry Recipes

Grilled Lemon Herb Chicken

Ingredients:
4 boneless, skinless chicken breasts
1/4 cup fresh lemon juice
2 tablespoons olive oil
2 cloves garlic, minced
1 teaspoon dried oregano
1 teaspoon dried thyme
Salt and pepper to taste
Lemon wedges for garnish

Preparation Method:
In a bowl, whisk together lemon juice, olive oil, minced garlic, oregano, thyme, salt, and pepper to create the marinade.

Put the chicken breasts inside a resealable plastic bag or shallow dish and pour the marinade on them. Ensure the chicken is evenly coated. Marinate in the refrigerator for at least 30 minutes, or preferable, overnight for additional flavor.

Preheat the grill to medium-high heat.

Take out the chicken from the marinade and let excess to drain out. Discard the used marinade.

Grill the chicken for 6-8 minutes per side, or until the internal temperature reaches 165°F (74°C) and the chicken is cooked through.

Allow the grilled chicken to rest for a few minutes before serving. Garnish with lemon wedges.

Nutritional Value (Per Serving):
Calories: 250
Protein: 30g
Fat: 11g
Carbohydrates: 3g
Fiber: 1g
Sugars: 0g
Sodium: 350mg

Spicy Turkey and Quinoa Stuffed Peppers

Ingredients:
4 big bell peppers, halved, with seeds removed
1 pound lean ground turkey
1 cup cooked quinoa

1 can (15 oz) of black beans, drained and rinsed
1 cup corn kernels (fresh or frozen)
1 cup diced tomatoes
1 teaspoon ground cumin
1 teaspoon chili powder
1/2 teaspoon smoked paprika
Salt and pepper to taste
1 cup shredded cheese (optional, for topping)
Fresh cilantro or green onions for garnish

Preparation Method:
Preheat the oven to 375°F (190°C).

In a large skillet, brown the ground turkey over medium heat until fully cooked. Drain any excess fat.

Add cooked quinoa, black beans, corn, diced tomatoes, ground cumin, chili powder, smoked paprika, salt, and pepper to the skillet. Mix well and cook for an additional 5 minutes until flavors meld.

Put the bell pepper halves in a baking tray.

Spoon the turkey and quinoa mixture into each pepper half, pressing down gently to pack the filling.

If desired, place shredded cheese on top of each filled pepper.

Cover the baking dish with foil and bake for 25-30 minutes, or until peppers are tender.

Remove the foil and bake for an additional 5-10 minutes to melt the cheese and achieve a golden brown top.

Before serving, garnish with chopped fresh cilantro or green onions.

Nutritional Value (per serving, assuming 4 servings):
Calories: ~350
Protein: ~25g
Carbohydrates: ~40g
Fiber: ~8g
Fat: ~10g
Saturated Fat: ~3g
Cholesterol: ~55mg
Sodium: ~400mg

Rosemary Garlic Beef Skewers

Ingredients:
1.5 lbs (680g) lean beef, cut into 1-inch cubes
2 tablespoons fresh rosemary, chopped
4 cloves garlic, minced
3 tablespoons olive oil
1 tablespoon balsamic vinegar
Salt and pepper to taste
Wooden or metal skewers (if using wood, soak them in water for 30 minutes)

Preparation Method:
In a bowl, combine the chopped rosemary, minced garlic, olive oil, balsamic vinegar, salt, and pepper to create the marinade.

Place the beef cubes in a resealable plastic bag or shallow dish and pour the marinade over them. Ensure the beef is evenly coated. Marinate in the refrigerator for at least 2 hours, preferably overnight for optimum flavor.

If using wooden skewers, thread the marinated beef cubes onto the soaked skewers.

Preheat the grill or grill pan to medium-high heat.

Grill the skewers for about 8-10 minutes, turning occasionally, or until the beef reaches your desired level of doneness.

Remove off the grill and allow the skewers to rest for a few minutes before serving.

Nutritional Value (per serving, assuming 4 servings):
Calories: ~300 kcal
Protein: ~35g
Fat: ~16g
Carbohydrates: ~2g
Fiber: ~0.5g
Sugars: ~0.5g
Sodium: ~80mg

Mediterranean Chicken Salad

Ingredients:
2 boneless, skinless chicken breasts
6 cups mixed salad greens
1 cup cherry tomatoes, halved
1 cucumber, sliced
1/2 cup kalamata olives, pitted
1/2 cup crumbled feta cheese
1/4 cup red onion, thinly sliced

2 tablespoons extra-virgin olive oil
1 tablespoon red wine vinegar
1 teaspoon dried oregano
Salt and pepper to taste
Lemon wedges for garnish

Preparation Method:
Season the chicken breasts with half of the dried oregano, salt and pepper.

Grill or pan-sear the chicken until fully cooked, approximately 6-8 minutes per side. Let it rest for a few minutes before slicing.

In a large bowl, combine the salad greens, cherry tomatoes, cucumber, olives, feta cheese, and red onion.

Whisk together the olive oil, red wine vinegar, and remaining dried oregano to create the dressing. Adjust salt and pepper to taste.

Place slices of grilled chicken on top of the salad.

Pour the dressing over the salad and gently toss to mix.

Garnish with lemon wedges for added flavor.

Serve immediately and enjoy the vibrant flavors of the Mediterranean.

Nutritional Value (per serving):
Calories: 350
Protein: 30g
Carbohydrates: 10g
Fat: 20g
Fiber: 4g
Vitamin C: 35% of daily recommended intake
Calcium: 15% of daily recommended intake
Iron: 20% of daily recommended intake

Lean Bison Chili

Ingredients:
1 lb lean ground bison
1 onion, diced
2 bell peppers (any color), diced
3 cloves garlic, minced
1 can (15 oz) drained and rinsed black beans
1 can (15 oz) drained and rinsed kidney beans
1 can (28 oz) crushed tomatoes
1 cup low-sodium beef broth
2 tablespoons chili powder
1 tablespoon cumin
1 teaspoon smoked paprika
1 teaspoon oregano
Salt and pepper to taste

Optional toppings: shredded cheese, Greek yogurt, green onions

Preparation Method:
In a large pot over medium heat, brown the lean ground bison, breaking it apart with a spatula as it cooks.

Add in the diced onions, bell peppers, and minced garlic to the pot. Sauté until the vegetables are tender.

Pour in crushed tomatoes and beef broth, stirring to combine.

Add black beans, kidney beans, chili powder, cumin, smoked paprika, oregano, salt, and pepper. Mix well.

Bring the chili to a simmer, then reduce the heat to low and let it cook for at least 30 minutes to allow flavors to meld.

Adjust seasoning if needed and serve hot. Top with shredded cheese, a dollop of Greek yogurt, or green onions if desired.

Nutritional Value (per serving, approximately 1 cup):
Calories: 250
Protein: 25g
Fat: 8g
Carbohydrates: 20g
Fiber: 6g
Sugar: 5g
Sodium: 500mg

Herb-Crusted Baked Chicken Breast

Ingredients:
4 boneless, skinless chicken breasts
1 cup breadcrumbs
2 tablespoons fresh parsley, finely chopped
1 tablespoon fresh thyme, minced
1 teaspoon dried oregano
1 teaspoon garlic powder
Salt and pepper to taste
2 tablespoons olive oil
1 tablespoon Dijon mustard

Preparation Method:
Preheat your oven to 400°F (200°C).

In a shallow bowl, combine breadcrumbs, chopped parsley, minced thyme, dried oregano, garlic powder, salt, and pepper. Mix well.

In a separate bowl, whisk together olive oil and Dijon mustard.

Dip each chicken breast into the olive oil and mustard mixture, ensuring it's evenly coated.

Press each chicken breast into the herb and breadcrumb mixture, ensuring the crust adheres well on both sides.

Lay the coated chicken breasts on a baking sheet covered with parchment paper.

Bake in the preheated oven for 20-25 minutes or until the internal temperature reaches 165°F (74°C) and the crust is golden brown.

Let the chicken rest for a few minutes before serving.

Nutritional Value (per serving):
Calories: approximately 250 kcal
Protein: 30g
Carbohydrates: 15g

Fat: 8g
Fiber: 2g
Sugars: 1g
Sodium: 400mg

Garlic Ginger Stir-Fried Beef with Broccoli

Ingredients:
1 pound flank steak, thinly sliced
2 cups broccoli florets
3 cloves garlic, minced
1 tablespoon fresh ginger, grated
2 tablespoons soy sauce (low-sodium)
1 tablespoon oyster sauce
1 tablespoon sesame oil
2 tablespoons vegetable oil
1 teaspoon cornstarch
1/4 cup beef broth
1 tablespoon rice vinegar
1 teaspoon honey
Optional: Sesame seeds and green onions for garnish

Preparation Method:
In a bowl, mix the sliced flank steak with soy sauce, oyster sauce, and cornstarch. Let it marinade for at least 15 minutes.

Heat up the vegetable oil in a wok or big skillet over medium-high heat. Add minced garlic and grated ginger, sauté for 1-2 minutes until fragrant.

Add the marinated beef to the wok and stir-fry until browned and cooked through. Remove the beef from the wok and set aside.

In the same wok, add a bit more oil if needed and stir-fry broccoli florets until they are tender-crisp, about 3-4 minutes.

In a small bowl, whisk together beef broth, sesame oil, rice vinegar, and honey. Pour the sauce over the broccoli in the wok.

Return the cooked beef to the wok, toss everything together until well-coated and heated through.

If preferred, garnish with sesame seeds and chopped green onions.

Nutritional Value (per serving, serves 4):
Calories: 320
Protein: 25g
Carbohydrates: 10g
Fiber: 3g

Sugars: 3g
Fat: 20g
Saturated Fat: 5g
Cholesterol: 60mg
Sodium: 650mg
Potassium: 520mg
Vitamin A: 15%
Vitamin C: 90%
Calcium: 4%
Iron: 20%

Turkey and Sweet Potato Hash

Ingredients:
1 pound lean ground turkey
2 medium sweet potatoes, peeled and diced
1 onion, finely chopped
1 bell pepper, diced
2 cloves garlic, minced
1 teaspoon smoked paprika
1 teaspoon ground cumin
Salt and pepper to taste
2 tablespoons olive oil
Fresh parsley for garnish (optional)

Preparation Method:
Heat up the olive oil in a big skillet over medium-high heat.

Add the ground turkey, breaking it apart with a spatula, and cook until browned.

Add the diced sweet potatoes to the skillet and cook for about 5 minutes, stirring occasionally, until they start to soften.

Stir in the chopped onion, bell pepper, and minced garlic. Cook for another 5-7 minutes or until the vegetables are soft.

Sprinkle smoked paprika, ground cumin, salt, and pepper over the mixture. Stir well to combine.

Continue cooking for another 5 minutes, allowing the flavors to meld and the sweet potatoes to fully cook.

Taste and adjust seasonings if necessary.

Garnish with fresh parsley if desired before serving.

Nutritional Value (Per Serving - Serves 4):
Calories: 320
Protein: 22g
Carbohydrates: 25g
Dietary Fiber: 4g
Sugars: 7g

Fat: 15g
Saturated Fat: 3g
Cholesterol: 60mg
Sodium: 120mg
Vitamin A: 160% DV
Vitamin C: 70% DV
Iron: 15% DV

Lemon Dill Roasted Chicken Thighs

Ingredients:
4 bone-in, skin-on chicken thighs
2 tablespoons olive oil
2 tablespoons fresh lemon juice
2 cloves garlic, minced
1 tablespoon fresh dill, chopped
1 teaspoon lemon zest
Salt and pepper to taste

Preparation Method:
Preheat the oven to 400°F (200°C).

In a small bowl, whisk together olive oil, lemon juice, minced garlic, chopped dill, lemon zest, salt, and pepper to create the marinade.

Place the chicken thighs in a zip-top bag or shallow dish and pour the marinade over them, ensuring each piece is well-coated. Marinate in the refrigerator for at least 30 minutes to allow the flavors to integrate.

Remove the chicken from the refrigerator and let it come to room temperature for about 15 minutes.

Place the chicken thighs on a baking sheet lined with parchment paper or a lightly oiled baking dish.

Roast in the preheated oven for 35-40 minutes or until the chicken reaches an internal temperature of 165°F (74°C) and the skin is golden and crispy.

Garnish with additional fresh dill and lemon slices if desired before serving.

Nutritional Value (per serving):
Calories: 300 kcal
Protein: 25g
Fat: 20g
Carbohydrates: 2g
Fiber: 0.5g
Sugars: 0.5g
Sodium: 400mg

Quinoa and Turkey Stuffed Acorn Squash

Ingredients:
2 acorn squash, halved and seeds removed
1 cup quinoa, rinsed
2 cups lean ground turkey
1/2 cup dried cranberries
1/4 cup chopped fresh parsley
1 teaspoon dried thyme
1 teaspoon ground cumin
Salt and pepper to taste
Olive oil for drizzling

Preparation Method:
Preheat the oven to 375°F (190°C).

Place the acorn squash halves on a baking sheet, cut sides down. Bake for 30-40 minutes or until the squash is soft.

While the squash is baking, cook quinoa according to package instructions.

In a large skillet, brown the ground turkey over medium heat until fully cooked. Drain any excess fat.

In a bowl, combine cooked quinoa, ground turkey, dried cranberries, parsley, thyme, cumin, salt, and pepper. Mix well.

Once the squash halves are done baking, flip them over and fill each half with the quinoa and turkey mixture.

Drizzle olive oil over the stuffed squash.

Return the stuffed squash to the oven and bake for an additional 15-20 minutes or until the filling is heated through and the tops are slightly crispy.

Nutritional Value (per serving, assuming 4 servings):
Calories: 450
Protein: 28g
Carbohydrates: 56g
Dietary Fiber: 9g
Sugars: 16g
Fat: 14g
Saturated Fat: 3g
Cholesterol: 70mg
Sodium: 120mg
Vitamin C: 30% DV
Iron: 25% DV
Calcium: 8% DV

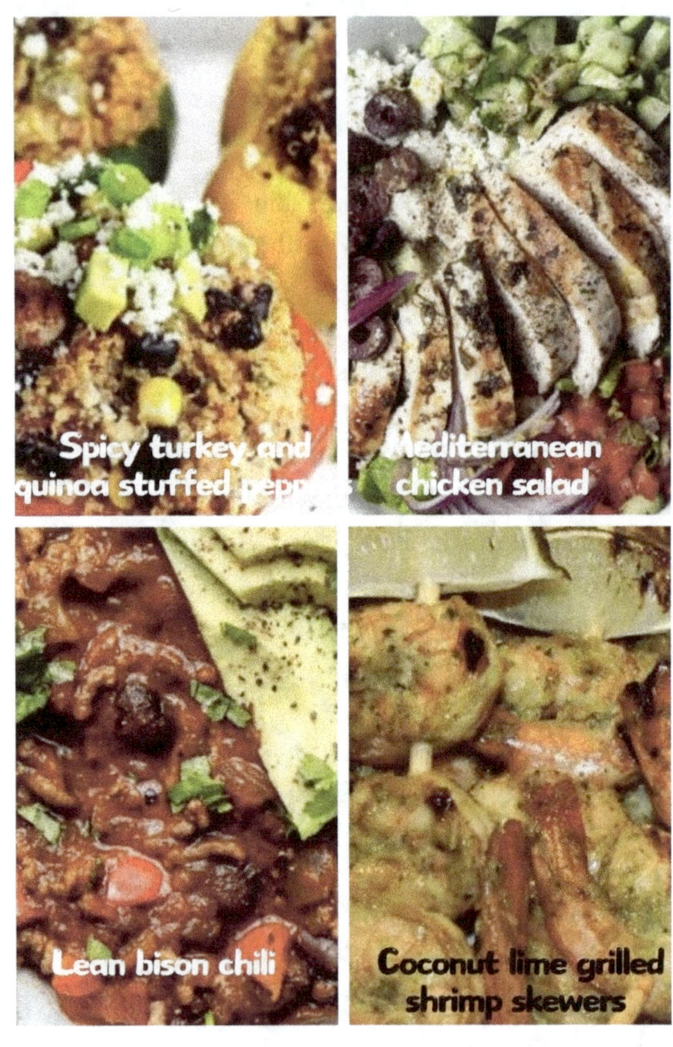

Spicy turkey and quinoa stuffed peppers
Mediterranean chicken salad
Lean bison chili
Coconut lime grilled shrimp skewers

Chapter 5: Pasta and Soup Recipes

Quinoa Linguine with Roasted Vegetables

Ingredients:
8 oz quinoa linguine
2 cups mixed vegetables (bell peppers, cherry tomatoes, zucchini, and red onion), diced
3 tablespoons olive oil
3 cloves garlic, minced
1 teaspoon dried oregano
1 teaspoon dried basil
Salt and pepper to taste
Grated Parmesan cheese for serving (optional)

Preparation Method:
Preheat the oven to 400°F (200°C).

In a large bowl, toss the mixed vegetables with 2 tablespoons of olive oil, minced garlic, dried oregano, dried basil, salt, and pepper.

Place the seasoned vegetables on a baking sheet in a single layer.

Roast the vegetables in the preheated oven for about 20-25 minutes or until they are soft and slightly caramelized.

While the vegetables are roasting, cook the quinoa linguine according to package instructions. Drain and set aside.

In a large skillet, heat the remaining 1 tablespoon of olive oil. Add the roasted vegetables and cooked quinoa linguine to the skillet. Toss to combine and heat through.

Serve the quinoa linguine with roasted vegetables hot, optionally topped with grated Parmesan cheese.

Nutritional Value (per serving):
Calories: 380 kcal
Protein: 10g
Carbohydrates: 55g
Fiber: 8g
Fat: 15g
Saturated Fat: 2g
Cholesterol: 0mg
Sodium: 120mg

Lentil Pasta with Spinach and Cherry Tomatoes

Ingredients:
8 oz (about 225g) lentil pasta
2 cups fresh spinach, washed and chopped
1 pint cherry tomatoes, halved
3 cloves garlic, minced
2 tablespoons olive oil
1/4 teaspoon red pepper flakes (optional)
Salt and pepper to taste
Freshly grated Parmesan cheese for garnish (optional)

Preparation Method:
Cook the lentil pasta according to package instructions. Drain and set aside.

In a large pan, heat up the olive oil over medium heat. Add in the minced garlic and sauté until aromatic.

Add cherry tomatoes to the pan and cook for 3-5 minutes, allowing them to soften.

Toss in the chopped spinach and cook until wilted.

Combine the cooked lentil pasta with the vegetables in the pan. Mix well.

If desired, season with salt, pepper, and red pepper flakes. Stir to combine.

Serve the Lentil Pasta with Spinach and Cherry Tomatoes hot, garnished with freshly grated Parmesan cheese if desired.

Nutritional Value (per serving):
Calories: 350
Protein: 15g
Carbohydrates: 45g
Fiber: 8g
Sugars: 4g
Fat: 12g
Saturated Fat: 2g
Cholesterol: 0mg
Sodium: 300mg

Zucchini Noodles in Tomato Basil Sauce

Ingredients:
4 medium-sized zucchinis, spiralized into noodles
2 cups cherry tomatoes, halved
3 cloves garlic, minced

1 can (14 oz) crushed tomatoes
1/4 cup fresh basil, chopped
2 tablespoons olive oil
Salt and pepper to taste
Optional: Grated Parmesan cheese for garnish

Preparation Method:
Heat up the olive oil in a big skillet over medium heat.

Add minced garlic and sauté until fragrant.

Add in the cherry tomatoes and cook until they begin to soften.

Pour in the crushed tomatoes, stirring to combine. Simmer for 10-15 minutes.

Season with salt and pepper, adjusting to your preferred taste.

Add zucchini noodles to the skillet, tossing them in the sauce until just tender.

Stir in fresh basil and cook for an additional 2 minutes.

Remove from heat and serve the zucchini noodles with tomato basil sauce.

Optionally, garnish with grated Parmesan cheese.

Nutritional Value (per serving):
Calories: 150
Protein: 5g
Carbohydrates: 20g
Dietary Fiber: 6g
Sugars: 12g
Fat: 7g
Saturated Fat: 1g
Cholesterol: 0mg
Sodium: 400mg

Chickpea Penne with Broccoli and Lemon Garlic Sauce

Ingredients:
2 cups chickpea penne pasta
3 cups broccoli florets
2 tablespoons olive oil
3 cloves garlic, minced
1 teaspoon lemon zest
2 tablespoons fresh lemon juice
Salt and pepper to taste
Red pepper flakes (optional for added heat)
1/4 cup grated Parmesan cheese (optional as garnish)

Fresh parsley, chopped (for garnish)

Preparation Method:
Cook the chickpea penne pasta according to package instructions. Drain and set aside.

In a big pan, heat up the olive oil over medium heat. Add in the minced garlic and sauté until fragrant.

Add broccoli florets to the pan and sauté for 5-7 minutes, or until they are tender-crisp.

Toss the cooked chickpea penne into the pan with the broccoli, combining them evenly.

In a small bowl, whisk together lemon zest, lemon juice, salt, pepper, and red pepper flakes if desired.

Pour the lemon garlic sauce over the pasta and broccoli, stirring well to coat.

Cook for another 2-3 minutes, allowing the flavors to infuse.

Serve the Chickpea Penne with Broccoli hot, garnished with Parmesan cheese and fresh parsley if desired.

Nutritional Value (per serving):
Calories: 380 kcal
Protein: 15g
Carbohydrates: 50g
Dietary Fiber: 10g
Sugars: 4g
Fat: 14g
Saturated Fat: 2g
Cholesterol: 5mg
Sodium: 280mg

Whole Wheat Spaghetti with Kale Pesto and Cherry Tomatoes

Ingredients:
8 oz whole wheat spaghetti
2 cups kale, stemmed and chopped
1/2 cup fresh basil leaves
1/3 cup grated Parmesan cheese
1/3 cup walnuts, toasted
2 cloves garlic, minced
1/2 cup extra-virgin olive oil
Salt and pepper to taste
1 cup cherry tomatoes, halved

Preparation Method:
Cook the whole wheat spaghetti according to package instructions, then drain and set aside.

In a food processor, combine kale, basil, Parmesan, toasted walnuts, and minced garlic.

Pulse the ingredients while slowly drizzling in the olive oil until a smooth pesto consistency is achieved.

Season the pesto with salt and pepper to taste, adjusting as needed.

Toss the cooked spaghetti with the kale pesto until well coated.

Gently fold in the halved cherry tomatoes.

Serve immediately, garnished with extra Parmesan and a sprinkle of fresh basil if desired.

Nutritional Value (per serving, serves 4):
Calories: 420
Protein: 12g
Fat: 25g
Carbohydrates: 42g
Fiber: 8g
Sugars: 3g

Sodium: 180mg

Butternut Squash and Lentil Soup

Ingredients:
1 medium-sized butternut squash, peeled and diced
1 cup of dried green or brown lentils, rinsed
1 onion, finely chopped
2 carrots, peeled and diced
2 celery stalks, diced
3 cloves garlic, minced
1 teaspoon ground cumin
1 teaspoon ground coriander
1/2 teaspoon smoked paprika
6 cups vegetable broth
Salt and pepper to taste
2 tablespoons olive oil
Fresh parsley for garnish

Preparation Method:
In a big pot, heat up the olive oil over medium heat. Add chopped onion, garlic, carrots, and celery. Sauté until the vegetables are softened.

Stir in ground cumin, ground coriander, and smoked paprika. Cook for an additional 2 minutes to enhance flavors.

Add diced butternut squash, lentils, and vegetable broth to the pot. Bring to a boil, then reduce heat and simmer until lentils and squash are tender (usually around 20-25 minutes).

Season with salt and pepper to taste.

Using an immersion blender, partially blend the soup to create a creamy texture while leaving some chunks.

Garnish with fresh parsley before serving.

Nutritional Value (per serving - serves 4):
Calories: 280
Protein: 14g
Carbohydrates: 50g
Fiber: 12g
Sugars: 6g
Fat: 4g
Saturated Fat: 1g
Cholesterol: 0mg
Sodium: 800mg

Quinoa Minestrone with Mixed Vegetables

Ingredients:
1 cup quinoa, rinsed
1 can (15 oz) of kidney beans, drained and rinsed
1 cup diced carrots
1 cup diced zucchini
1 cup diced celery
1 cup diced tomatoes
1/2 cup green beans, chopped
1/2 cup chopped onion
3 cloves garlic, minced
6 cups vegetable broth
2 teaspoons olive oil
1 teaspoon dried oregano
1 teaspoon dried basil
Salt and pepper to taste
Fresh parsley for garnish

Preparation Method:
In a big pot, heat up the olive oil over medium heat. Add garlic and onions, sauté until fragrant.

Add carrots, zucchini, celery, green beans, and tomatoes. Cook for about 5-7 minutes until vegetables begin to soften.

Pour in vegetable broth, kidney beans, oregano, basil, salt, and pepper. Bring to a boil.

Add quinoa to the pot, reduce heat to low, cover, and simmer for 15-20 minutes or until quinoa is cooked.

Adjust seasoning if needed. Serve hot, garnished with fresh parsley.

Nutritional Value (per serving, assuming 4 servings):
Calories: 350
Protein: 15g
Carbohydrates: 60g
Fiber: 12g
Fat: 5g
Saturated Fat: 1g
Cholesterol: 0mg
Sodium: 800mg
Potassium: 950mg

Sweet Potato and Black Bean Chili

Ingredients:
2 medium sweet potatoes, peeled and diced

1 can (15 oz) drained and rinsed black beans
1 can (15 oz) diced tomatoes, undrained
1 cup corn kernels (fresh or frozen)
1 onion, finely chopped
3 cloves garlic, minced
1 bell pepper, diced
1 jalapeño, finely chopped (adjust for spice preference)
1 tablespoon olive oil
2 teaspoons ground cumin
2 teaspoons chili powder
1 teaspoon smoked paprika
Salt and pepper to taste
4 cups vegetable broth
Fresh cilantro and lime wedges for garnish

Preparation Method:
In a big pot, heat up the olive oil over medium heat. Add chopped onion, garlic, bell pepper, and jalapeño. Sauté until softened.

Add in the ground cumin, chili powder, and smoked paprika. Cook for another minute until aromatic.

Add diced sweet potatoes, black beans, diced tomatoes, corn, and vegetable broth. Bring to a boil, then lower the heat and simmer until sweet potatoes are soft.

Season with salt and pepper to taste. Simmer for an additional 15-20 minutes to let flavors meld.

Garnish with fresh cilantro and lime wedges then serve hot.

Nutritional Value (per serving, assuming 4 servings):
Calories: 320
Protein: 10g
Fat: 5g
Carbohydrates: 60g
Fiber: 12g
Sugars: 10g
Vitamin A: 400% DV
Vitamin C: 90% DV
Iron: 15% DV
Calcium: 8% DV

Barley and Mushroom Soup with Thyme

Ingredients:
1 cup pearl barley
2 tablespoons olive oil
1 onion, finely chopped
2 cloves garlic, minced
8 oz (about 225g) mushrooms, sliced

2 carrots, diced
2 celery stalks, diced
6 cups vegetable broth
1 teaspoon dried thyme
Salt and pepper to taste
Fresh parsley for garnish

Preparation Method:
Rinse the pearl barley under cold water and set aside.

In a big pot, heat up the olive oil over medium heat. Add the chopped onion and garlic, sauté until softened.

Add the sliced mushrooms, diced carrots, and celery to the pot. Cook for about 5-7 minutes until the vegetables are soft.

Pour in the vegetable broth and add the rinsed pearl barley to the pot.

Season with dried thyme, salt, and pepper. Bring the soup to a boil, then reduce the heat to simmer and cover. Let it cook for about 30-40 minutes or until the barley is tender.

Adjust seasoning if needed. Scoop soup into dishes and garnish with fresh parsley.

Nutritional Value (per serving - serves 4):
Calories: approximately 250
Protein: 8g
Carbohydrates: 48g
Fiber: 10g
Fat: 5g
Sodium: 800mg

Spinach and White Bean Soup with Whole Grain Farro

Ingredients:
1 cup whole grain farro, soaked and drained
1 can (15 oz) drained and rinsed white beans
4 cups fresh spinach, washed and chopped
1 onion, finely chopped
2 carrots, diced
2 celery stalks, diced
3 cloves garlic, minced
6 cups vegetable broth
2 tablespoons olive oil
1 teaspoon dried thyme
Salt and pepper to taste
Optional: Parmesan cheese for garnish

Preparation Method:
In a big pot, heat up the olive oil over medium heat. Add chopped onions, carrots, and celery. Saute until vegetables are softened.

Add in the minced garlic and cook for an additional minute until aromatic.

Pour in vegetable broth and bring to a simmer.

Add soaked and drained farro to the pot. Simmer for about 15-20 minutes or until the farro is tender.

Stir in white beans and continue simmering for an additional 5 minutes.

Add chopped spinach and dried thyme. Cook until the spinach wilts and the soup is heated through.

Season with salt and pepper to taste.

Serve hot, optionally garnished with Parmesan cheese.

Nutritional Value (per serving):
Calories: 320
Protein: 12g
Carbohydrates: 55g

Fiber: 12g
Fat: 7g
Saturated Fat: 1g
Cholesterol: 0mg
Sodium: 800mg

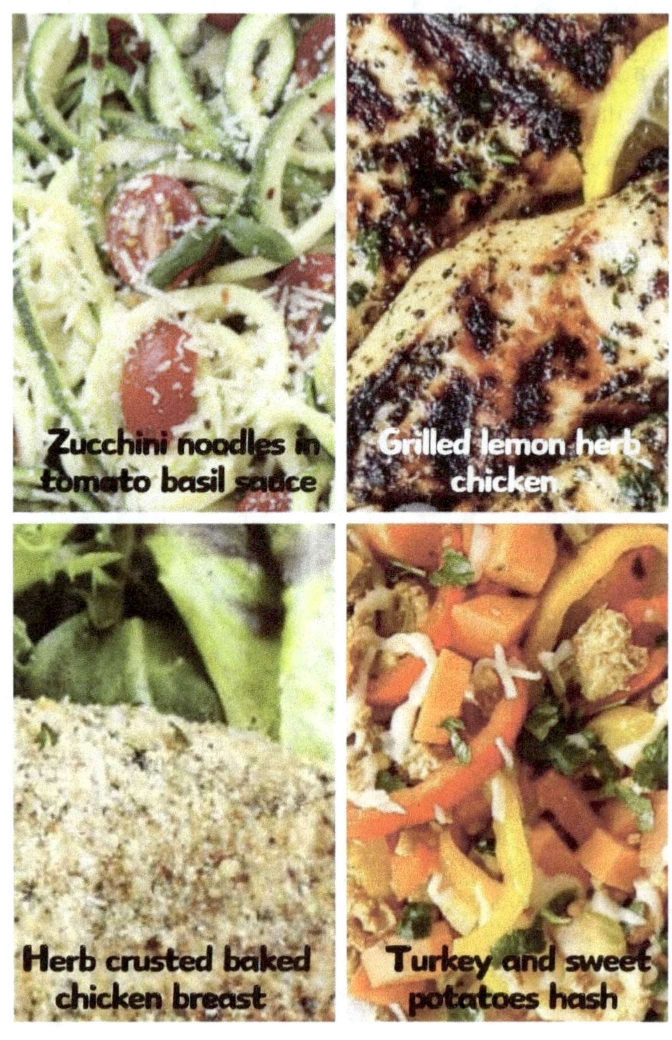

Zucchini noodles in tomato basil sauce
Grilled lemon herb chicken
Herb crusted baked chicken breast
Turkey and sweet potatoes hash

Chapter 6: Salad Recipes

Quinoa Power Salad

Ingredients:
1 cup quinoa (rinsed and cooked)
2 cups mixed greens
1 cup cherry tomatoes (halved)
1 cucumber (diced)
1/2 red onion (finely sliced)
1 avocado (diced)
1/2 cup feta cheese (crumbled)

For the Lemon Vinaigrette:
1/4 cup extra virgin olive oil
2 tablespoons fresh lemon juice
1 teaspoon Dijon mustard
Salt and pepper to taste

Preparation Method:
Cook quinoa according to the instructions on the package and let it cool.

In a large bowl, combine the cooked quinoa, mixed greens, cherry tomatoes, cucumber, red onion, avocado, and feta cheese.

In a small bowl, whisk together the ingredients for the Lemon Vinaigrette until well combined.

Drizzle the vinaigrette on the salad and mix gently to coat all ingredients evenly.

Nutritional Value (per serving):
Calories: 400
Protein: 12g
Carbohydrates: 35g
Fiber: 8g
Sugars: 4g
Fat: 25g
Saturated Fat: 6g
Cholesterol: 20mg
Sodium: 350mg

Mediterranean Chickpea Salad

Ingredients:
1 can (15 oz) drained and rinsed chickpeas
1 cup cherry tomatoes, halved
1/2 cup Kalamata olives, sliced
1 red bell pepper, diced
1/2 red onion, finely chopped
1 cucumber, diced

1/2 cup crumbled feta cheese

3 tablespoons extra virgin olive oil

2 tablespoons red wine vinegar

1 teaspoon dried oregano

Salt and pepper to taste

Preparation Method:

In a large bowl, combine chickpeas, cherry tomatoes, Kalamata olives, red bell pepper, red onion, cucumber, and feta cheese.

In a small bowl, mix together the olive oil, red wine vinegar, dried oregano, salt, and pepper.

Pour the dressing over the salad and toss gently to combine, ensuring all ingredients are evenly coated.

Refrigerate for at least 30 minutes before serving to allow flavors to infuse.

Serve chilled and garnish with additional feta cheese if desired.

Nutritional Value (Per Serving - Serves 4):

Calories: 280

Protein: 8g

Carbohydrates: 23g

Fiber: 6g

Sugars: 5g
Fat: 18g
Saturated Fat: 5g
Cholesterol: 15mg
Sodium: 480mg

Kale and Berry Bliss Salad

Ingredients:
4 cups kale, finely chopped
1 cup mixed berries (blueberries, strawberries, raspberries)
1/2 cup walnuts, chopped
1/2 cup goat cheese, crumbled
1/4 cup balsamic vinaigrette dressing

Preparation Method:
Wash and dry the kale thoroughly, then remove the stems and finely chop the leaves.

In a large salad bowl, combine the chopped kale with the mixed berries.

Toast the chopped walnuts in a dry skillet over medium heat until lightly golden, then let them cool.

Add the toasted walnuts and crumbled goat cheese to the salad.

Pour the balsamic vinaigrette dressing on the salad ingredients.

Toss the salad gently to ensure an even distribution of ingredients and dressing.

Nutritional Value (per serving):
Calories: 300
Protein: 10g
Carbohydrates: 20g
Dietary Fiber: 5g
Sugars: 8g
Fat: 22g
Saturated Fat: 6g
Cholesterol: 15mg
Sodium: 200mg

Spicy Shrimp and Avocado Salad

Ingredients:
1 pound of large shrimp, peeled and deveined
6 cups mixed greens
1 ripe avocado, diced
1 cup cherry tomatoes, halved
1 cup canned black beans, drained and rinsed

1 cup corn kernels (fresh or thawed if frozen)
1/4 cup chopped fresh cilantro
1 lime, juiced
2 tablespoons olive oil
1 teaspoon ground cumin
1/2 teaspoon smoked paprika
1/4 teaspoon cayenne pepper (adjust to taste)
Salt and pepper to taste

Preparation Method:
In a bowl, combine shrimp with olive oil, cumin, smoked paprika, cayenne pepper, salt, and pepper. Toss to coat evenly.

Heat a skillet over medium-high heat. Cook shrimp for 2-3 minutes per side or until opaque and cooked through. Remove from heat.

In a large salad bowl, assemble the mixed greens, diced avocado, cherry tomatoes, black beans, corn, and cilantro.

Add the cooked shrimp on top of the salad.

In a small bowl, whisk together lime juice and olive oil. Drizzle the dressing over the salad.

Gently mix the salad to combine all the ingredients.

Serve immediately, and enjoy the vibrant flavors!

Nutritional Value (per serving, approximate):
Calories: 350 kcal
Protein: 25g
Fat: 18g
Carbohydrates: 25g
Fiber: 8g
Sugar: 3g
Vitamin C: 30% DV
Iron: 15% DV
Calcium: 8% DV

Sweet Potato and Quinoa Harvest Salad

Ingredients:
1 cup quinoa, cooked
2 medium-sized sweet potatoes, peeled and diced
2 cups arugula
1/2 cup pecans, toasted
1/2 cup dried cranberries
Salt and pepper to taste

Orange Maple Dressing:
1/4 cup orange juice
2 tablespoons maple syrup

2 tablespoons extra virgin olive oil
1 tablespoon apple cider vinegar
1 teaspoon Dijon mustard
Salt and pepper to taste

Preparation Method:
Preheat your oven to 400°F (200°C).

Mix the diced sweet potatoes with olive oil, salt, and pepper. Roast in the oven for about 20-25 minutes or until soft and slightly caramelized.

In a large bowl, combine cooked quinoa, arugula, roasted sweet potatoes, toasted pecans, and dried cranberries.

In a small bowl, whisk together the orange juice, maple syrup, olive oil, apple cider vinegar, Dijon mustard, salt, and pepper to create the dressing.

Drizzle the dressing over the salad and toss gently to coat all ingredients evenly.

Serve chilled or at room temperature.

Nutritional Value (per serving):
Calories: 350 kcal
Protein: 8g

Carbohydrates: 55g

Dietary Fiber: 7g

Sugars: 18g

Fat: 12g

Saturated Fat: 1.5g

Cholesterol: 0mg

Sodium: 120mg

Asian Sesame Ginger Chicken Salad

Ingredients:

1 lb grilled chicken breast, sliced

6 cups Napa cabbage, shredded

1 cup mandarin oranges, peeled and segmented

1 cup snap peas, thinly sliced

1 cup carrots, julienned

2 tablespoons sesame seeds

Dressing:

3 tablespoons soy sauce

2 tablespoons sesame oil

1 tablespoon rice vinegar

1 tablespoon honey

1 teaspoon fresh ginger, grated

1 clove garlic, minced

Preparation Method:

In a large bowl, combine the shredded Napa cabbage, grilled chicken slices, mandarin oranges, snap peas, and julienned carrots.

In a small bowl, whisk together the dressing ingredients: soy sauce, sesame oil, rice vinegar, honey, grated ginger, and minced garlic.

Drizzle the dressing on the salad and mix until all the ingredients are well coated.

Sprinkle sesame seeds on top for an added crunch.

Serve immediately, or refrigerate for a refreshing chilled salad.

Nutritional Value (per serving):

Calories: 350 kcal
Protein: 30g
Carbohydrates: 20g
Dietary Fiber: 5g
Sugars: 10g
Fat: 18g
Saturated Fat: 3g
Cholesterol: 70mg
Sodium: 700mg

Caprese Salad with a Twist

Ingredients:
Heirloom tomatoes, sliced
Fresh mozzarella, sliced
Fresh basil leaves
Pine nuts, toasted
Balsamic glaze
Extra virgin olive oil

Preparation Method:
Arrange slices of heirloom tomatoes and fresh mozzarella on a serving platter, alternating them.

Tuck fresh basil leaves in between the tomato and mozzarella slices.

Sprinkle toasted pine nuts over the salad.

Drizzle balsamic glaze and extra virgin olive oil over the salad.

Optionally, season with a pinch of salt and black pepper to taste.

Nutritional Value (per serving):
Calories: Approx. 220 kcal
Protein: 12g

Fat: 16g
Carbohydrates: 10g
Fiber: 2g
Sugar: 5g

Tuna and White Bean Delight

Ingredients:
1 can (about 5 oz) of tuna, drained
1 can (15 oz) drained and rinsed cannellini beans
1 cup cherry tomatoes, halved
1/4 cup red onion, finely chopped
2 cups arugula
2 tablespoons fresh lemon juice
2 tablespoons extra virgin olive oil
Salt and pepper to taste

Preparation Method:
In a large mixing bowl, combine the drained tuna, cannellini beans, cherry tomatoes, and chopped red onion.

In a small bowl, whisk together the fresh lemon juice and extra virgin olive oil to create the dressing.

Pour the dressing over the tuna and bean mixture, gently tossing to coat the ingredients evenly.

Place a bed of arugula on serving plates.

Spoon the tuna and bean mixture over the arugula.

Season with salt and pepper to taste.

Garnish with fresh herbs like parsley or dill for additional flavor (optional).

Nutritional Value (per serving):
Calories: ~380 kcal
Protein: ~30g
Carbohydrates: ~30g
Fiber: ~8g
Fat: ~15g
Omega-3 fatty acids from tuna contribute to heart health, while beans provide fiber for digestive wellness. Arugula adds vitamins and minerals, creating a balanced and nutritious meal.

Roasted Veggie and Quinoa Delight

Ingredients:
1 cup quinoa, rinsed
2 cups mixed vegetables (zucchini, bell peppers, cherry tomatoes), chopped

1/2 cup feta cheese, crumbled
2 tablespoons olive oil
Salt and pepper to taste
Fresh basil leaves for garnish

Preparation Method:
Preheat the oven to 400°F (200°C).

Combine the quinoa with 2 cups of water in a saucepan. Allow to a boil, then lower the heat, cover, and simmer for 15 minutes or until quinoa is well cooked and water is absorbed.

While the quinoa is cooking, pour the chopped vegetables on a baking sheet. Drizzle with olive oil, salt and pepper, then mix to coat. Roast in the preheated oven for about 20 minutes or until vegetables are tender and slightly caramelized.

In a big bowl, add together the cooked quinoa and roasted vegetables. Toss gently to mix.

Sprinkle crumbled feta cheese over the quinoa and roasted vegetables.

Transfer the salad to a serving dish. Garnish with fresh basil leaves.

Optional Dressing:
You can drizzle the salad with a light vinaigrette or a squeeze of lemon for added flavor.

Nutritional Value (Per Serving):
Calories: ~350 kcal
Protein: ~12g
Carbohydrates: ~45g
Dietary Fiber: ~7g
Sugars: ~5g
Fat: ~15g
Saturated Fat: ~5g
Cholesterol: ~20mg
Sodium: ~300mg

Greek-Inspired Cauliflower Salad

Ingredients:
1 medium cauliflower, cut into florets
1 cup cherry tomatoes, halved
1 cucumber, diced
1/2 cup Kalamata olives, sliced
1/2 cup crumbled feta cheese
1/4 cup red onion, finely chopped
Fresh parsley, chopped (for garnish)

Lemon Oregano Dressing:
1/4 cup extra virgin olive oil
2 tablespoons lemon juice
1 teaspoon dried oregano
Salt and pepper to taste

Preparation Method:
Preheat the oven to 400°F (200°C).

Toss cauliflower florets with a drizzle of olive oil, salt, and pepper. Roast in the oven for about 20-25 minutes or until golden brown and soft.

In a large mixing bowl, combine roasted cauliflower, cherry tomatoes, cucumber, Kalamata olives, feta cheese, and red onion.

In a small bowl, whisk together the olive oil, lemon juice, dried oregano, salt, and pepper to create the dressing.

Pour the dressing over the salad and toss gently to coat all ingredients evenly.

Garnish with fresh parsley and additional feta if desired.

Refrigerate for at least 30 minutes before serving to allow flavors to infuse properly.

Nutritional Value (per serving, assuming 4 servings):
Calories: ~220
Protein: ~8g
Fat: ~18g
Carbohydrates: ~10g
Fiber: ~4g
Sugar: ~4g

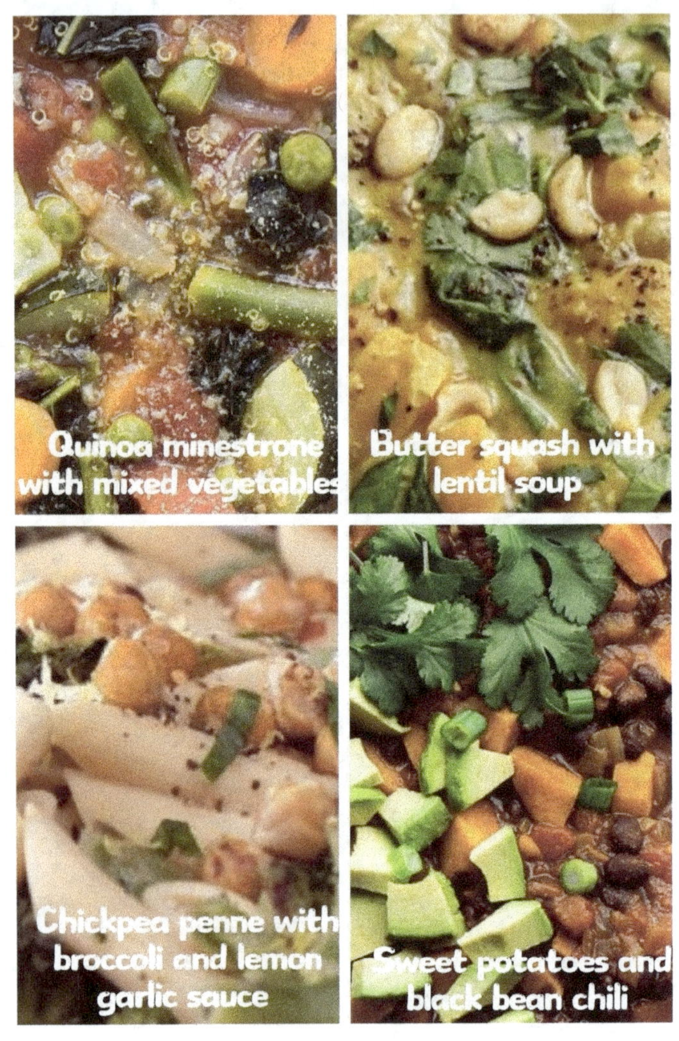
Quinoa minestrone with mixed vegetables
Butter squash with lentil soup
Chickpea penne with broccoli and lemon garlic sauce
Sweet potatoes and black bean chili

Conclusion

In conclusion, following the Endomorph Diet is more than simply a physical transformation; it is a genuine commitment to restoring your health and energy. As you've progressed through these pages, you've learned about customized nutrition and the importance of matching your dietary choices to your own body type.

Remember that the Endomorph Diet is not a restricted plan, but rather a guide for feeding your body in a way that complements its natural tendencies. It's about eating clean, nutrient-dense meals that boost your metabolism and improve your overall health. The route to good health is about progress rather than perfection. Celebrate little triumphs, such as inches gone, improved energy, or a restored sense of confidence.

Your dedication to this lifestyle goes beyond the limitations of a typical diet. It's a comprehensive strategy that combines diet, mindfulness, and self-care. Embrace the diversity of whole meals, taste the flavors, and relish the wonderful changes emerging inside you.

As you continue down this route, keep in mind that failures are a normal part of any transformative journey. Learn from them, adjust, and go ahead. Your body is a remarkable, adaptable mechanism, and the Endomorph Diet allows you to operate in harmony with it.

Finally, I want you to think of the Endomorph Diet as a long-term and empowering lifestyle, rather than a passing fad. Your improved understanding of nutrition and how it affects your specific body type gives you the skills you need to make educated decisions that align with your health objectives.
Accept this path with confidence, knowing that you have the knowledge, resilience, and capacity to transform your well-being. Your body is a unique vessel capable of transformation and rejuvenation. The Endomorph Diet is your guide to achieving its full potential. Here's to being healthier, happier, and more active.

21-Day Meal Plan

Day 1
Breakfast: Quinoa Power Bowl
Lunch: Grilled Lemon Herb Salmon
Dinner: Quinoa Linguine with Roasted Vegetables

Day 2
Breakfast: Sweet Potato and Spinach Omelette
Lunch: Mediterranean Chickpea Salad
Dinner: Spicy Turkey and Quinoa Stuffed Peppers

Day 3
Breakfast: Avocado Toast with Poached Eggs
Lunch: Shrimp and Quinoa Stir-Fry
Dinner: Butternut Squash and Lentil Soup

Day 4
Breakfast: Chia Seed Pudding Parfait
Lunch: Quinoa Power Salad
Dinner: Rosemary Garlic Beef Skewers

Day 5
Breakfast: Protein-Packed Smoothie Bowl
Lunch: Baked Cod with Mediterranean Salsa
Dinner: Lentil Pasta with Spinach and Cherry Tomatoes

Day 6
Breakfast: Salmon and Avocado Wrap
Lunch: Kale and Berry Bliss Salad
Dinner: Mediterranean Chicken Salad

Day 7
Breakfast: Egg White Vegetable Scramble
Lunch: Zesty Lime Cilantro Tilapia
Dinner: Quinoa Minestrone with Mixed Vegetables

Day 8
Breakfast: Greek Yogurt Parfait
Lunch: Spicy Shrimp and Avocado Salad
Dinner: Lean Bison Chili

Day 9
Breakfast: Cottage Cheese and Pineapple Bowl
Lunch: Herb-Crusted Mahi-Mahi
Dinner: Zucchini Noodles in Tomato Basil Sauce

Day 10
Breakfast: Almond Butter Banana Pancakes
Lunch: Sweet Potato and Quinoa Harvest Salad
Dinner: Herb-Crusted Baked Chicken Breast

Day 11
Breakfast: Vegetable Frittata
Lunch: Cajun Blackened Catfish

Dinner: Chickpea Penne with Broccoli and Lemon Garlic Sauce

Day 12
Breakfast: Oatmeal with Nut Butter and Berries
Lunch: Mango Avocado Tuna Salad
Dinner: Garlic Ginger Stir-Fried Beef with Broccoli

Day 13
Breakfast: Whole Grain Breakfast Burrito
Lunch: Asian Sesame Ginger Chicken Salad
Dinner: Whole Wheat Spaghetti with Kale Pesto and Cherry Tomatoes

Day 14
Breakfast: Berry and Spinach Smoothie
Lunch: Coconut-Lime Grilled Shrimp Skewers
Dinner: Sweet Potato and Black Bean Chili

Day 15
Breakfast: Quinoa Power Bowl
Lunch: Lemon Dill Zucchini Noodles with Crab
Dinner: Turkey and Sweet Potato Hash

Day 16
Breakfast: Sweet Potato and Spinach Omelette
Lunch: Caprese Salad with a Twist
Dinner: Lemon Dill Roasted Chicken Thighs

Day 17
Breakfast: Avocado Toast with Poached Eggs
Lunch: Tuna and White Bean Delight
Dinner: Quinoa and Turkey Stuffed Acorn Squash

Day 18
Breakfast: Chia Seed Pudding Parfait
Lunch: Grilled Lemon Herb Chicken
Dinner: Barley and Mushroom Soup with Thyme

Day 19
Breakfast: Protein-Packed Smoothie Bowl
Lunch: Roasted Veggie and Quinoa Delight
Dinner: Grilled Lemon Herb Salmon

Day 20
Breakfast: Salmon and Avocado Wrap
Lunch: Greek-Inspired Cauliflower Salad
Dinner: Spicy Garlic Ginger Scallop Stir-Fry

Day 21
Breakfast: Egg White Vegetable Scramble
Lunch: Mediterranean Chicken Salad
Dinner: Spinach and White Bean Soup with Whole Grain Farro

www.ingramcontent.com/pod-product-compliance
Lightning Source LLC
Chambersburg PA
CBHW070847250726
48662CB00003B/1410